Healing Chest Pain

A Health Guide On Chest Pain Relief, Symptoms, Causes, Treatment, Medications

Dr. Nicholas Paul

Table of Contents

Chapter One 3

   Chest Pain 3

Chapter Two 13

   What are reasons chest ache? .. 13

Chapter Three 23

   What is the remedy for chest ache? 23

Chapter Four 32

   Pleuritis or pleurisy 32

Chapter Five 44

   Pneumonia 44

Chapter Six 55

Angina and coronary heart assault (myocardial infarction) 55

Chapter Seven 70

Aorta and aortic dissection......70

Chapter One

Chest Pain

What have to you recognized approximately chest ache?

Chest ache is one of the maximum not signs and symptoms that deliver an person to the emergency department. Seeking instant care can be lifesaving, and great public schooling has been undertaken to get sufferers to be searching for hospital therapy while chest ache strikes. You can be concerned which you are having a coronary heart assault; however there are numerous different reasons of ache within the chest that the medical doctor will don't forget. Some diagnoses of chest ache are existence threatening, at the same time as others are much less dangerous.

What reasons chest aches?

Deciding the motive of chest ache is now and again very hard and can require blood checks, X-rays, CT scans and different checks to type out the analysis. Often though, a cautious records taken via way of means of the medical doctor can be all this is wished.

There are many reasons of chest ache, and at the same time as many aren't serious, it could be hard to differentiate a coronary heart assault, pulmonary embolus, or aortic dissection, from any other analysis that isn't always existence threatening, like heartburn. For that reason, people are robotically suggested to are searching for scientific assessment for maximum sorts of chest ache.

What are the signs and symptoms of chest ache?

While every motive of chest ache has conventional signs and symptoms and symptoms and symptoms, there are sufficient versions in signs and symptoms that it could take particular checking out to attain a analysis. Tests to diagnose chest ache will rely on your present day fitness and outcomes of any checks or procedures.

Treatment for chest ache relies upon at the motive. Always are searching for hospital therapy in case you are having chest ache.

Chest Pain Symptoms

Chest ache may be related to signs and symptoms together with dizziness, lightheadedness, shortness of breath, or stabbing or burning sensations.

What are the distinct places of chest ache?

The following anatomic places can all be ability reasserts of chest ache:

The chest wall together with the ribs, the muscle groups, and the skin

The returned together with the spine, the nerves, and the returned muscle groups

The lung, the pleura (the liner of the lung), or the trachea

The coronary heart together with the pericardium (the sac that surrounds the coronary heart)

The aorta

The esophagus

The diaphragm, the flat muscle that separates the chest and belly cavities

Referred ache from the belly hollow space together with organs just like the belly, gallbladder, and pancreas, in addition to inflammation from the bottom of the diaphragm because of contamination, bleeding, or different sorts of fluid.

There can be conventional shows of symptoms and symptoms and signs and symptoms for lots illnesses however they also can gift atypically and there can also be full-size overlap a number of the signs and symptoms of every circumstance. Age, gender, and race can have an effect on presentation and the fitness care expert have to don't forget many variables earlier than achieving a analysis.

What are different signs and symptoms of chest ache?

Other symptoms and symptoms and symptoms that arise with chest ache consist of chest (coronary heart) ache, chest pain that consists of stress, squeezing, heaviness, or burning. Sometimes you could sense like you're choking or brief of breath. People who've had extreme chest ache describe it as pain that levels from sharp to dull, and generally, is placed within the jaw, neck, shoulders, upper stomach, and palms.

Signs like tension and different situations, exertion, eating, publicity to cold, or emotional pressure can motive tightness if the chest.

Chapter Two

What are reasons chest ache?

Pain may be because of nearly each shape within the chest. Different organs can produce distinct sorts of ache; unfortunately, the ache isn't always particular to every motive. Many motives can motive chest ache, for example:

Broken or bruised ribs

Pleuritis or pleurisy

Pneumothorax

Shingles

Pneumonia

Pulmonary embolus

Angina

Heart assault (myocardial infarction)

Pericarditis

The aorta and aortic dissection

The esophagus and reflux esophagitis

Referred belly ache

What are the danger elements for reasons of chest ache?

Coronary heart disorder

Smoking

High blood stress

High ldl cholesterol

Diabetes

Family records

Pulmonary embolus (blood clot to the lung)

Prolonged state of no activity together with mattress rest, lengthy vehicle or plane trips

Recent surgical treatment

Fractures

Birth manipulate tablet use (in particular if the affected person smokes cigarettes)

Cancer

Aortic dissection

High blood stress

Marfan syndrome

Ehlers-Danlos syndrome

Polycystic kidney disorder

Cocaine use

Pregnancy

What methods and checks diagnose the motive of chest ache?

The key to analysis is the affected person's scientific records. Learning approximately the character of the ache will provide the fitness care expert route as to what are affordable diagnoses to don't forget, and what are affordable to exclude. Understanding the high-satisfactory and amount of the ache, its related signs and symptoms and the affected person's danger elements for particular disorder, can assist the medical doctor investigate the opportunity of every ability motive and make selections approximately what diagnoses have to be taken into consideration and which of them may be discarded.

Differential analysis is a notion manner that healthcare experts use to don't forget after which get rid of ability reasons of an infection. As greater records are gathered, from both records, bodily exam, or checking out, the ability analysis listing is narrowed till the very last solution is achieved. Moreover, the affected person's reaction to healing interventions can enlarge or slim the differential analysis listing. In sufferers with chest ache, many feasible situations can be gift, and the fitness care expert will need to first don't forget the ones which are existence threatening. Using laboratory and X-ray checks might not be important to exclude doubtlessly deadly illnesses like coronary heart assault, pulmonary embolus, or aortic dissection while scientific capabilities and judgment are employed.

The affected person can be requested numerous inquiries to assist the fitness care expert recognize the high-satisfactory and amount of the ache. Patients use distinct phrases to explain ache, and it's far critical that the fitness care expert get an correct influence of the situation. The questions can also be requested in distinct ways.

The man or woman can be requested to give an explanation for their solution due to the fact now and again phrases suggest something distinct to different human beings. If the man or woman says that, "they aren't having chest ache," however they forget to inform the medical doctor that they may be feeling "chest stress." People might also additionally describe the ache as sharp, however they suggest excessive, at the same time as the medical doctor might imagine that sharp equals stabbing. The medical doctor's know-how of the high-satisfactory of ache is an critical first step in making the analysis.

There is a difference distinction among features of ache. The medical doctor wishes to recognize the kind of ache, and what sort of ache the man or woman is experiencing.

Chapter Three

What is the remedy for chest ache?

Treatment for chest ache relies upon at the motive.

Broken or bruised ribs

Readers Comments three Share Your Story

Bruised or damaged ribs are not accidents. Symptoms of damaged or bruised ribs consist of:

tenderness over the page of damage;

a damaged rib can be palpated (the fitness care expert can sense the rib fracture circulate while pressed);

the ache has a tendency to be Pleuritis (it hurts to take a deep breath and may be related to shortness of breath); and

due to the fact the encompassing muscle groups cross into spasm, there may be ache with any motion of the trunk.

The medical doctor will concentrate to the chest to ensure

that there may be no related lung harm. Sometimes, subcutaneous emphysema may be felt with a collapsed lung (pneumothorax), a sensation of feeling rice krispies while air leaks into the skin. A chest X-ray can be finished to search for a pneumothorax or pulmonary contusion (a bruised lung). Special X-rays seeking out rib fracture aren't wished for the reason that presence or absence of a fracture will now no longer modify the remedy plan or healing time. Special interest may be given to the top stomach for the reason that ribs guard the spleen and liver, to ensure there aren't anyt any related accidents.

The principal hassle of rib accidents is pneumonia. The lungs paintings like bellows. Normally, while one takes a breath, the ribs swing out and the diaphragm actions down, sucking air into the lungs. Because it hurts to take a deep breath, this mechanism is altered, and the lung underlying the damage might not absolutely enlarge due to the fact the affected person can't tolerate the ache. The end result is stagnant air and lung tissue that doesn't absolutely enlarge, inflicting a ability breeding floor for a lung contamination (pneumonia).

Rib damage remedy might also additionally consist of:

Pain manipulate with anti inflammatory medicines like ibuprofen and narcotic ache medicines to permit deep breaths to arise.

Application of ice to the affected vicinity and to periodically deep take breaths. An incentive pyrometer can be supplied to assist visualize the quantity of breath to take.

Ribs are now no longer wrapped or taped to assist with comfort. Wrapping damaged ribs decreases the cappotential of the lung beneath the injured vicinity to absolutely enlarge, which will increase the danger of growing pneumonia.

Whether damaged or bruised, rib accidents take three to six weeks to heal.

Chest Pain

See an in depth scientific example of the coronary heart plus our whole scientific gallery of human anatomy and physiology

Costochondritis

Occasionally, the joints and cartilage wherein ribs connect to the sternum (breastbone) might also additionally turn out to be infected. The ache has a tendency to arise with a deep breath, and there may be tenderness that may be felt while the edges of the sternum are palpated or touched. If there may be swelling and irritation related to the tenderness, it's far called Tietze's syndrome.

The maximum common motive for Costochondritis is idiopathic or unknown, that means there may be no cause of the ache. Other reasons consist of trauma to the vicinity, contamination (regularly viral), and fibromyalgia.

Though painful, the signs and symptoms remedy with symptomatic care, together with ice and/or heat compresses and anti inflammatory medicines (for example, ibuprofen). As with different chest wall ache, healing might also additionally take weeks. Taking deep breaths to save you the danger of pneumonia could be very critical.

Chapter Four

Pleuritis or pleurisy

The lung slides alongside the chest wall while a deep breath is taken. Both surfaces have a skinny lining referred to as the pleura to permit this sliding to arise. On occasion, viral infections can motive the pleura to turn out to be infected, after which in place of sliding smoothly, the 2 linings scrape in opposition to every different, inflicting ache. This kind of chest ache hurts with a deep breath, and feels just like the ache of pleurisy.

Viral infections are a not motive of pleurisy, even though there are numerous different infectious reasons together with tuberculosis. Other illnesses that may inflame the pleura consist of:

collagen vascular illnesses like sarcoidosis and systemic lupus erythematosus,

most cancers,

kidney failure,

rheumatoid arthritis,

headaches of radiation remedy,

headaches of chemotherapy, and headaches of surgical treatment.

The bodily examination can be rather unremarkable; however a friction rub can be heard over the page of pleural irritation. If a full-size quantity of fluid leaks from the irritation, the distance among the lung and the chest wall (the pleural area) can fill with fluid, called an effusion. When listening with a stethoscope, there can be reduced air access within the lung. As well, percussion, wherein the fitness care expert faucets at the chest wall like a drum, might also additionally monitor dullness of 1 aspect as compared to the different.

Often a chest X-ray is finished to evaluate the lung tissue and the presence or absence of fluid within the pleural hollow space.

Pleurisy is generally handled with an anti inflammatory medicine. This will regularly deal with an effusion as well. If the effusion is huge and is inflicting shortness of breath, thoracentesis (thora=chest + centesis=chickening out fluid) can be finished. For thoracentesis, a needle is located within the pleural area and the fluid withdrawn. Aside from making the affected person sense better, the fluid can be despatched for laboratory evaluation to assist with analysis. Ultrasound can be ordered, relying at the affected person's situation.

Pneumothorax

The lung is held in opposition to the chest wall via way of means of bad stress within the pleura. If this seal is damaged, the lung can cut back down, or crumble (called pneumothorax). This can be related to a rib damage or it could arise spontaneously. However, generally visible in folks that are tall and skinny, different danger elements for a collapsed lung consist of emphysema or asthma. Small blebs or vulnerable spots within the lung can wreck and motive the air leak that breaks the bad stress seal.

The not presentation is the intense onset of sharp chest ache related to shortness of breath, without a previous infection or warning. Physical exam exhibits reduced air access at the affected aspect. Percussion might also additionally display elevated resonance with tapping. Chest X-ray confirms the analysis.

Treatment relies upon what number of the lung is collapsed. If it's far a small quantity and crucial symptoms and symptoms are strong with a ordinary O2 sat, the pneumothorax can be allowed to enlarge on its personal with near monitoring. If there may be a bigger crumble, a chest tube might also additionally must be located into the pleural area via the chest wall to suck the air out and re-set up the bad stress. On occasion, thoracoscopy (thoraco=chest +scopy=see with a camera) can be taken into consideration to discover the bleb and to staple it shut. For greater, please examine the Pneumothorax article.

Tension pneumothorax is a rather uncommon existence-threatening occasion regularly related to trauma. Instead of a easy crumble of the lung, a situation can exist wherein the broken lung tissue acts as a one-manner valve permitting air to go into the pleural area however now no longer permitting it to escape. The pneumothorax length will increase with every breath and may save you blood from returning to the coronary heart and permitting the coronary heart to pump it returned to the body. If now no longer corrected quick with placement of a chest tube to alleviate tension, it is able to be deadly.

Shingles

Shingles is because of the varicella zoster virus, the equal one which reasons chickenpox. Once the virus enters the body, it hibernates within the nerve roots of the spinal column, handiest to emerge someday within the destiny. The rash is diagnostic because it follows the nerve root because it leaves the returned, and circles to the front of the chest, however by no means crosses the midline.

Once the rash appears, the analysis is rather smooth for the fitness care expert. Unfortunately, the ache of shingles might also additionally start some days earlier than the rash emerges and may be puzzling to each affected person and fitness care expert, for the reason that ache and burning might also additionally appear out of share to the findings on bodily exam.

The remedy for shingles consists of antiviral medicines like acyclovir (Zovirax) in conjunction with ache manipulates medicine. The ache from the infected nerve may be may be pretty extreme. Some sufferers might also additionally broaden postherpetic neuralgia, or persistent ache from the infected nerve, which might also additionally persist lengthy after the contamination, has cleared. Varieties of ache manipulate techniques are to be had from medicine to ache stimulators to surgical treatment.

Chapter Five

Pneumonia

Pneumonia is an contamination of the lung. In pneumonia, irritation can motive fluid buildup inside a phase of the lung tissue, lowering its cappotential to switch oxygen from air to the bloodstream.

Typical signs and symptoms of infectious pneumonia consist of:

Fever

Chills

Malaise

Other symptoms and symptoms and signs and symptoms consist of:

Cough,

Shortness of breath, and

Sputum production (coughing up mucus).

The maximum not reasons of a lung infections are because of Streptococcal pneumonia or Pneumococcus micro organism. The conventional presentation of a lung contamination because of the micro organism Streptococcal pneumonia or Pneumococcus, is acute onset of shaking chills, fever, and a cough that produces rusty brown sputum.

The medical doctor will test the affected person's crucial symptoms and symptoms (for abnormalities regular with an contamination), pulse and breathing rate, fever, and paying attention to chest sounds. To diagnose infectious pneumonia methods and check might also additionally consist of, a chest X-ray, blood checks, or elevated lactic acid (lactate). Treatment generally is with antibiotics.

Pulmonary embolism

A blood clot to the lung may be deadly and is one of the diagnoses that have to continually be taken into consideration while a affected person affords with chest ache.

The conventional symptoms and symptoms and signs and symptoms of a blood clot within the lung are ache while taking a deep breath, shortness of breath, and coughing up blood (hemoptysis); however greater generally, sufferers may have greater diffused signs and symptoms, and the analysis can be without difficulty missed.

Risk elements for pulmonary embolus consist of:

Prolonged state of no activity like an extended experience in a vehicle or plane

Recent surgical treatment or fracture

Birth manipulate pills (in particular related to smoking)

Cancer

Pregnancy

Thrombophilia (thrombo=clot + philia= attraction) accommodates a bunch of blood clotting disorders, which locations sufferers at danger for pulmonary embolism.

The pulmonary embolus starts off evolved in veins someplace else within the body, generally the legs, though it is able to arise within the pelvis, palms, or the principal veins within the stomach. When a thrombus or blood clot bureaucracy, it has the ability to interrupt free (now referred to as an embolus) and go with the flow downstream, returning to the coronary heart. The embolus can retain its adventure via the coronary heart after which can be pumped into the pulmonary circulate system, ultimately turning into lodged in one of the branches of the pulmonary artery and slicing off blood deliver to a part of the lung. This reduced blood glide would not permit sufficient blood to select out up oxygen within the lung, and the affected person can turn out to be markedly brief of breath.

As noted previously, the not court cases consist of:

Pleuritis chest ache from the infected lung

Bloody sputum,

Shortness of breath

The affected person also can have tension and sweat profusely. Depending upon the dimensions of the clot, the preliminary presentation can be fainting (syncope) or surprise wherein the affected person collapses, with reduced blood stress and adjusted intellectual function.

Depending at the severity of the embolus and the quantity of lung tissue at danger, the affected person might also additionally gift seriously ill (in extremis) with markedly unusual crucial symptoms and symptoms, or might also additionally seem alternatively ordinary. Physical exam might not be beneficial, and the diagnostic research is finished upon scientific suspicion primarily based totally on records and danger elements.

The analysis can be made immediately with imaging of the lungs or circuitously via way of means of locating a clot someplace else within the body. The approach used to make a analysis will rely on every person affected person's situation, however there are a few well-known equipment to be had, for example, D-Dimer, CT scans, ultrasound, angiography, and medicines.

Chapter Six

Angina and coronary heart assault (myocardial infarction)

The challenge for maximum sufferers and fitness care experts is that any chest ache might also additionally originate from the coronary heart. Angina is the time period given to ache that takes place due to the fact the coronary arteries (blood vessels to the coronary heart muscle) slim and reduces the quantity of oxygen that may be introduced to the coronary heart itself. This can motive the conventional signs and symptoms of chest stress or tightness with radiation to the arm or jaw related to shortness of breath and sweating.

Unfortunately, many human beings do not gift with conventional signs and symptoms, and the ache can be hard to explain -- or in a few human beings might not also be gift. Instead of angina or ordinary chest stress, their anginal equivalent (symptom they get in place of chest ache) can be indigestion, shortness of breath, weakness, dizziness, and malaise. Women and the aged are at better danger for having an extraordinary presentation of coronary heart ache.

The narrowing of blood vessels or atherosclerosis is because of plaque buildup. Plaque is a tender amalgam of ldl cholesterol and calcium that bureaucracy alongside the internal lining of the blood vessel and steadily decreases the diameter of the blood vessel and restricts the glide of blood. If the plaque ruptures, it is able to motive a blood clot to shape and absolutely block the vessel.

When a coronary artery absolutely occludes (turns into blocked), the muscle it substances blood to is liable to dying. This is a coronary heart assault or myocardial infarction. In maximum circumstances, this ache is greater excessive than ordinary angina, however again, there are numerous versions in symptoms and symptoms and signs and symptoms.

The analysis of angina is a scientific one. After the fitness care expert takes a cautious records and assesses the ability danger elements, the analysis is both fairly pursued in any other case it's far taken into consideration now no longer to be gift. If angina is the ability analysis, similarly assessment might also additionally consist of electrocardiograms (EKG or ECG) and blood checks.

Treatment of angina

The cause of creating the analysis of angina is to repair ordinary blood deliver to coronary heart muscle earlier than a coronary heart assault takes place and everlasting muscle harm outcomes. Aside from minimizing danger elements via way of means of controlling blood stress, ldl cholesterol, and diabetes, and preventing smoking, medicines may be used to make the coronary heart beat greater efficiently (for example, beta blockers), to dilate blood vessels (for example, nitroglycerin) and to make blood much less probable to clot (aspirin).

Treatment of coronary heart assault

An acute coronary heart assault (myocardial infarction) is a real emergency considering that entire blockage of blood deliver will motive a part of the coronary heart muscle to die and get replaced via way of means of scar tissue. This lessens the cappotential of the coronary heart to pump blood to fulfill the body's wishes. As well, injured coronary heart muscle is irritable and may motive electric disturbances like ventricular fibrillation, a circumstance wherein the coronary heart jiggles like Jell-O and can't beat in a coordinated fashion. This is the motive of unexpected loss of life in coronary heart assault. The motive of an acute coronary heart assault is the rupture of a ldl cholesterol plaque in a coronary artery. This reasons a blood clot to shape and occlude the artery.

The remedy for coronary heart assault is emergent recuperation of blood deliver. Two alternatives consist of use of a drug like TPA or TNK to dissolve the blood clot (thrombolytic remedy) or emergency coronary heart catheterization and the usage of a balloon to open up the blocked vicinity (angioplasty) and maintaining it open with a mesh cage referred to as a stent. Emergent angioplasty is desired if the affected person lives near a sanatorium with that functionality however many human beings do now no longer. Staged handled with preliminary thrombolytic remedy observed via way of means of angioplasty is likewise affordable.

Coronary artery skip surgical treatment is taken into consideration while there may be diffuse artery disorder that isn't always amenable to angioplasty and stenting.

Pericarditis

The coronary heart is contained in a sac referred to as the pericardium. Just like in pleurisy, this sac can turn out to be infected and motive ache. As against angina, this ache has a tendency to be sharp and is because of the infected sac rubbing in opposition to the outer layers of the coronary heart.

The maximum not motive of pericarditis both is a viral infection or is unknown (idiopathic). Inflammatory illnesses of the body (rheumatoid arthritis, systemic lupus erythematosus), kidney failure, and most cancers are different situations that may motive pericarditis. Trauma, in particular from steerage wheel accidents in motor car injuries also can motive pericarditis and doubtlessly inflicting blood to build up within the skinny pericardial sac.

The ache with pericarditis is excessive, sharp, has a tendency to be worse while mendacity down, and is relieved via way of means of leaning forward. Because the ache may be so extreme, radiate to the arm or neck, and motive a few shortness of breath, it's far now and again wrong for angina, pulmonary embolus, or aortic dissection. Associated signs and symptoms might also additionally consist of fever and malaise relying upon the motive.

History is beneficial in making the analysis, seeking out a current viral infection, and asking approximately beyond scientific records. Physical exam might also additionally monitor a friction rub while paying attention to the coronary heart sounds.

The electrocardiogram might also additionally display modifications regular with pericarditis, however on occasion; the EKG might also additionally mimic an acute coronary heart assault.

Echocardiogram is beneficial if there may be fluid within the pericardial sac related to the irritation.

An anti inflammatory medicine like ibuprofen is the remedy for pericarditis. Addressing the underlying motive may also direct remedy.

Cardiac tapenade is a hassle of pericarditis. Pressure from extra fluid constructed up within the pericardial sac is so super that it prevents blood from returning to the coronary heart. The analysis is made clinically the usage of the triad of (Beck's triad):

Low blood stress

Distention of neck veins

Muffled coronary heart tones

Treatment calls for setting a needle into the pericardium to withdraw fluid and/or surgical treatment to open a window within the pericardium to save you destiny fluid buildup.

Chapter Seven

Aorta and aortic dissection

The aorta is the huge blood vessel that exits the coronary heart and can provide blood to the body. It consists of layers of muscle that want to be sturdy sufficient to resist the stress generated via way of means of the thrashing coronary heart. In a few human beings, a tear can arise in one of the layers of the aortic wall, and blood can music among the wall muscle groups. This is referred to as an aortic dissection, and is doubtlessly existence threatening.

The kind of dissection and remedy relies upon wherein within the aorta the dissection takes place. Type A dissections are placed within the ascending aorta, which runs from the coronary heart to the aortic arch wherein blood vessels that deliver the mind and palms exit. Type B dissections are placed within the descending aorta that runs via the chest and down into the stomach.

The majority of aortic dissections arise as an extended-time period outcome of poorly managed excessive blood stress. Other related situations consist of:

Marfan's syndrome

Trauma

Pregnancy

A past due post-operative hassle of open coronary heart surgical treatment

The ache from aortic dissection takes place all of sudden and regularly is defined as excessive, stabbing, or ripping. It can be constant, or the ache can be Pleuritis (worse with a deep breath). Often it radiates to the returned. Often, if the dissection takes place within the chest, it could be pressured with the ache of coronary heart assault, esophagitis, or pericarditis. If the aortic dissection is placed close to of beneath the diaphragm, it is able to mimic renal colic (ache from a kidney stone).

Diagnosis is primarily based totally upon records, evaluate of the danger elements, bodily exam, and scientific suspicion. Physical exam might also additionally monitor loss or put off of pulses within the wrist or leg while evaluating one aspect to the different. A new coronary heart murmur can be detected if the dissection entails the aortic valve that connects the aorta with the coronary heart. If blood vessels exiting the aorta are worried within the vicinity of dissection, the organs that they deliver can be at danger. Stroke and paralysis may be visible in dissection. Blood deliver may be misplaced to kidneys and bowel and/or to palms and legs.

The analysis of aortic dissection is showed via way of means of imaging, maximum generally via way of means of CT angiography of the aorta. Echocardiography or ultrasound can also be used to picture the aorta.

Type A dissections of the ascending aorta are handled via way of means of surgical treatment wherein the broken piece of aorta is eliminated and changed with an synthetic graft. Sometimes the aortic valve wishes to be repaired or changed if it's far broken.

Type B dissections are to begin with handled via way of means of medicines to govern blood stress and keep it in a ordinary range. Beta blockers and calcium channel blocker medicines are generally used. If scientific remedy fails, surgical treatment can be important.

If the dissection tears absolutely via all 3 layers of the aortic wall, then the aorta ruptures. This is a catastrophe, and greater than 50% of affected sufferers die earlier than achieving a sanatorium. The universal mortality of aortic rupture is more than 80%.

Esophagus and reflux esophagitis

The esophagus is a muscular tube that consists of meals from the mouth to the belly. The decrease esophageal sphincter (LES) is a specialised band of muscle on the decrease cease of the esophagus that capabilities as a valve to hold belly contents from spilling returned into the esophagus. Should that valve fail, belly contents, together with acidic digestive juices, can reflux returned and aggravate the liner of the esophagus. While the belly has a shielding barrier lining to guard it from ordinary digestive juices, this safety is lacking within the esophagus.

Reflux esophagitis (additionally called GERD, gastro esophageal reflux disorder) can gift with burning chest and top belly ache that radiates to the throat and can be related to a bitter flavor within the returned of the throat referred to as water brash. It might also additionally gift after food or at bedtime while the affected person lies flat. There may be full-size spasm of the esophageal muscle groups, and the ache may be excessive. The ache of reflux esophagitis may be wrong for angina, and vice versa.

The bodily exam is generally now no longer beneficial, and a scientific analysis is regularly made without similarly checking out. Endoscopy can be accomplished to have a take a observe the liner of the esophagus and belly.

When signs and symptoms are lengthy-standing, they will be related to, or motive Barrett's esophagus (precancerous modifications affecting the cells lining the decrease esophagus). Manometer may be finished to degree stress modifications within the esophagus and belly to determine whether or not the LES is running appropriately. Barium swallow or astrograph with fluoroscopy is a kind of X-ray wherein the swallowing styles of the esophagus may be evaluated.

Treatment for reflux esophagitis consists of:

Dietary and way of life modifications to restriction the quantity of acid that may backsplash from the belly into the esophagus.

Elevating the pinnacle of the mattress lets in gravity to hold acid from refluxing.

Smaller meal sizes can restriction belly distention.

Caffeine, alcohol, anti inflammatory medicines, and

smoking are irritants to the liner of the belly and esophagus and have to be avoided.

Acid blockers like omeprazole (Prilosec) or lansoprazole (Prevacid) can lower the quantity of belly acid this is produced, and antacids like Maalox or Mylanta can assist bind extra acid.

The headaches of acid reflux disease disorder rely on its severity and its duration. Chronic reflux can motive modifications within the lining of the esophagus (Barrett's esophagus) which might also additionally result in most cancers. Reflux may deliver acid contents into the returned of the mouth into the larynx (voice box) and motive hoarseness or recurrent cough. Aspiration pneumonia may be because of acid and meals debris inhaled into the lung.

The End